KU-350-422

RAW FOOD TREATMENT OF CANCER

By
Kristine Nolfi, M.D.

TEACH Services, Inc.
Brushton, New York 12916

Published by

TEACH Services, Inc.
www.tsibooks.com

RAW FOOD TREATMENT
OF CANCER

RAW FOOD TREATMENT OF CANCER

Before I realized the actual importance of raw vegetable food, my attitude was exactly the same as that of other physicians—to treat the symptoms of the disease without thinking of preventing it. It ought to be the duty of the medical profession in future to find means of preventing to a much higher degree than now, instead of attempting to cure later on.

That I, as a physician, went in for exclusively raw vegetable food is due to the fact that I became ill, even seriously ill, myself. I developed cancer of the breast. The disease had, of course, been preceded by wrong nourishment and wrong habits in the course of my twelve years of hospital training, when I suffered from sluggish digestion and catarrh of the stomach all the time, disorders which are still of quite common occurrence among hospital staff members. Since that time no change of the hospital diet has taken place in Denmark in this very important domain. On one occasion I was in a dying condition because of a bleeding gastric ulcer. This made me abandon meat and fish, and I became a vegetarian. Later, I took to eating a good deal of raw vegetable food. In this manner my digestion became regulated, and I felt better, though not completely well. In the winter of 1940 to 1941 I was exceptionally tired and dull, but I was unable to ascertain any specific disease. At that time I did not understand what was wrong with me, but in the course of the spring I discovered a small node in my right breast.

I Discover My Cancer

Tired and dull as I was, I did not pay any attention to it until five weeks later. I discovered that the node was the size of a hen's egg. It had grown into the skin—a thing only cancer does. As a physician I had seen enough to be unwilling to submit to the treatment of cancer generally employed. I consulted my good friend, Dr. M. Hindhede, who dissuaded a trial microscopy. It would open up the bloodstreams and the cancer would spread; so I gave it up. And then I felt it as quite a natural thing that I would have to carry through a one hundred percent raw vegetable diet.

I went in search of nature, lived for some time on a small island in the Kattegat, took sun baths from four to five hours daily, slept in a tent, bathed several times a day, and lived exclusively on a raw vegetable diet. Later I introduced this habit of life at the sanatorium "Humlegaarden."

Improvement Realized After Two Months

But I was still tired and continued to be so for the first two months, and during that period the node in the breast did not diminish; it remained unchanged.

But then the improvement came. The node diminished, my strength returned, apparently I recovered and felt better than I had for many years. When I had experienced good health in this manner for about a year, I tried by way of experiment (and urged to do so by Dr. Hindhede) to revert to a vegetarian diet supplemented by fifty percent of raw vegetable food.

My Cancer Reoccurs on Cooked Food

But it was no good. In three to four months I began to feel a stinging pain in the breast, in the sore-like tissue which the cancer had left where it had originally adhered to the skin. The pain increased much during the weeks that followed, and I realized that the cancer had begun to develop again.

Cancer Under Control Again on Raw Food Diet

Once more I reverted to pure, raw food, which caused the pain to subside rapidly and the fatigue to become less pronounced. But, being a doctor, I realized that I would have to use the experience I had gained to help my sick fellow creatures. So I set up my home so that I could have four or five patients staying with me the next summer. We took one hundred percent raw vegetables as a diet, and all went well; but it was not satisfactory with so few patients. I understood that this cause would have to be advocated under quite different and larger conditions if any proofs were to be given. On my initiative a joint stock company was then formed which bought a property, "Humlegaarden." Well suited for the purpose it was set up as a sanatorium, where I became the chief physician. Here we eat only raw vegetable food, patients as well as employees, and the establishment is now in its sixth year.

Why Raw Foods Are Beneficial

Now, what is the reason why a one hundred percent raw vegetable diet exerts such a beneficial effect on civilized individuals? First and foremost, because the raw food is live food as it is handed to us by nature. We all know that life on earth is completely dependent on our sun. If we had no sun the earth would be without any life, dark and icy cold. Vital force is therefore identical with sun energy!

According to Dr. Hesselink, it is, however, only the plant with its widely unfolded thin green leaves, that is able to catch the sunlight and to deposit it in the form of roots and tubers, fruit and seeds. We human beings and the animals, with massive bodies, are not able to utilize it to a sufficiently high degree. Therefore both men and beast use plants as carriers between the sun and themselves. A fresh, raw vegetable diet is sunlight nourishment!

Dr. Bircher-Benner, of Zurich, realized this long ago. Dr. Hesselink, from Holland, believes that it is the atoms which are the carriers of the solar energy.

Raw Foods of Highest Nutritional Value

Fresh, raw vegetable food possesses the highest nutritive value, and this cannot be increased or improved; anything else, such as heating, drying, storing, fermentation or preservation, will reduce and destroy its value. Boiled vegetables taste of nothing, so something must be done to make them palatable. We mix many different things together; we add salt, sugar, spices and butter. We remove the germ and the husk from the wheat to use the flour for baking. We polish the rice, we refine the sugar, we remove the skin, seeds, and cores of apples and pears, we peel the potatoes and scrape the carrots. Meat, fish, eggs and cheese supply us with an enormous surplus of animal protein. We make beverages of coffee and cocoa beans and tea, which contain stimulating poisons.

Drug-Taking Is Widespread

We use the grapes for wine and brandy—intoxicating poisons—which first stimulate the grey cortex of the brain, and later paralyze it. We preserve food with chemicals, such as benzoic acid, salicylic acid, nitre, boric acid and sulfurous acid in order that it may keep well, and look attractive. Further, we take anodynes, hypnotics, sedatives and aperients—all strong chemical poisons—substances that are foreign to the organism. Among drugs which are misused to a great extent, tablets for headache, hypnotics and aperients are much too predominant. In a small country like Denmark the adviser on pharmacological matters of the Public Health Authorities is able to give us the following figures: consumption of drugs for headache—105 tons, aperients—15 tons, hypnotics—9 tons—annually.

Raw Food Way To Overcome Tobacco Habit

Nicotine, too, is a ruinous stimulant, a still stronger poison than spirits; it causes sclerosis of the heart and the cardiac musculature to become undernourished. The heart becomes a flaccid bag instead of a firm muscle. Many busy men about the age of fifty years die of heart failure caused by chronic nicotine poisoning. Here too, I have experienced that patients on a pure, raw vegetable diet gradually lose their taste for tobacco completely.

The ground, too, is wrongly cultivated when it is fertilized too much and too uniformly with chemical manure. We may run the risk that the ground becomes just as diseased as man—over acidified, over-nourished, and that it yields sick plants which are not fit for human food.

Raw Foods Easy to Digest

Raw food is termed live food by me, in contrast with such food as has been treated by heating, which I consider dead food. Care should be taken that the food does not include substances which counteract the chemistry of the organism, so that the waste products are not retained too long and putrefy in the large intestine. The best food is therefore completely natural food which has not been subjected to denaturation of any kind. To this must be added that live food is much easier to digest; it helps in the digestion itself just as the living baby cooperates in its delivery. Raw vegetables have been digested in the stomach and the intestines in an hour; boiled vegetables require almost three hours and leave more waste products, also offensive stools, impure blood, and poisoned and gradually impaired organs, whereas the raw food—live food, the sunlight nourishment, dissolves and excretes these poisons. Raw food is easy to digest, it spares and strengthens the organism in every respect because of its content of life, bases, and vitamins in their natural, living combination and relationship to one another. Everybody who can think must be able to understand that our present nutrition is highly destructive and is the most common and most serious cause of physical and psychic diseases and constitutional degeneration. We must seek more wholesome nourishment and more wholesome habits of life if we are to live better now and in the future. We cannot afford to compromise when life and health are concerned. We must follow the only right way—the 100% raw vegetable and fruit diet.

Let us consider for a moment how it influences our many different diseases. In the individual case it will always, on the one hand, depend on how good a constitution the patient has and how old he is, and on the other hand how poisoned, weakened and broken his constitution has gradually become because of preceding wrong nutrition and wrong habits. But it may be said, largely, that if, in spite hereof, the organism is fairly fit for work and able to utilize the exclusively raw diet, the latter will exert a curative effect on almost all our diseases, both those we have acquired during our span of life and those determined by hereditary predispositions.

Humankind Presently In a Degenerated State

Even the baby unborn may be injured in various ways. The impaired germ may determine both physical and psychic diseases. The baby may be injured by the wrong nutrition of the mother, because it is nourished through the impure blood of the mother. This may pave the way to disease so that the baby is born ill. After its birth the condition is aggravated, mostly because the mother's milk is not as good, both qualitatively and quantitatively. Children all over the civilized world are born weaklings in a mild or severe degree, and who can estimate the future consequence thereof? Therefore, the sooner we go in for exclusively raw vegetable food, the sooner that it will exert its effect. Children are assisted by nature, older individuals are rather opposed by nature. When a mother goes in for pure raw food, her milk secretion is immediately increased, the child thrives in all respects, the vitality is increased, and the mother can soon begin to give even young babies an addition of finely chopped fruit and vegetables; never, however, fruit and vegetables at the same time—always separately. It borders on the incomprehensible that a change can be effected so rapidly, just by giving the child wholesome mother's milk, as much as it requires, and afterwards, fruit and vegetables.

Raw Food Diet Humanizes Us

I have often experienced how a large family of brothers and sisters living exclusively on raw vegetables become healthy, happy, lively and nice children in the course of a few months, so good is the effect of the exclusively raw vegetable diet in childhood, which is still assisted by nature and has not yet been ruined. The effect does not appear quite as soon in adults, but it is indisputable that raw vegetables exert a good effect on adults too, even psychically—it brings about equanimity and harmony, kindness and sympathy.

But what of the elderly sick or the very sick people who have (,one in for this diet too late? How about them?

Raw Food Diet Helps All

Well, they have to be patient, energetic, and very interested, and they must be able to rest much, at any rate to begin with. The first few days may be troublesome until they have become accustomed to this different food and habit of life. But they will soon do better, the bowels open regularly—two to three times daily—and this is a great encouragement to many.

Raw vegetable food exerts an excellent effect on all forms of rheumatism and rheumatic arthritis when these diseases have not progressed too far. A good effect is also seen on the diseases related to loading with uric acid; it applies to psoriasis, hemicrania, stone-formation in the gall bladder, the renal pelvis and the urinary bladder. Almost all diseases of the skin are corrected, in many cases even rapidly. Loss of hair, fat formation, and dandruff cease. All infections are corrected or improved.

Women who carry through the raw diet during pregnancy feel well—delivery takes place rapidly and almost without pain, the slender, healthy strong baby cooperates. The raw food produces copious and good milk for the child during the first year if the mother continues with the diet.

7

Cancer is the terminal stage pathology: Here a one hundred percent raw vegetable diet may prove helpful, alleviate the pain, prolong the life to some extent, because it agrees well with the patient. In most favorable cases, when the cancer is dealt with in time, it may perhaps also be checked even for many years in some cases. I am an example of this myself, but then the seat of the cancer must not be in a vital organ, such as the lungs, liver or stomach. And treatment with raw food should be commenced as soon as the cancer is discovered, and it is an absolutely necessary condition that it is carried through one hundred percent.

I want now to tell a little about my own case from 1942 to the present year. Up to 1946 I was doing well on my exclusively raw diet—the cancer of the breast was completely quiescent, and my general health was good.

Dried Fruits Inferior To Fresh Fruits

But in the spring of 1946 we got some dried fruit from Sweden (raisins, dates, prunes and figs). I thought that it would be all right to eat, but it was not. These are the fruits which have been treated with chemical poisons in order to preserve them and to make them look attractive. Having taken them for three or four months I suddenly developed violent pains in the scar-like tissue of the breast, and on closer examination, I found a small node in the right breast, in the same place as before. Once more I reverted to the fresh raw food, and the node disappeared.

Biopsy Dangerous

The last and most dangerous thing for me was, however, the trial microscopy against which I had been dissuaded by Dr. M. Hindhede. I had to let it be done because of so many physicians maintaining that I had never suffered from cancer. It was made at the Radium Centre in Copenhagen in January 1948. The trial microscopy was positive; there were cancer cells in the scar-like tissue in the skin of the right breast, but it was a benign form called scirrhus. My originally malignant, rapidly growing form of cancer had thus, under the influence of raw food, been converted into a benign form of cancer, which remains quiescent. But still this interference was just on the point of stirring up the cancer so much as to frighten me seriously. For the first time I developed metastases (two small nod-

8

ules) in the armpit; and about six months —on the exclusively raw diet—were required to make them subside again. But it went well this time. Since then I have been in excellent health—all through last summer I was up at sunrise, and in my garden where I have been working hard several hours daily. This was far more wholesome than sitting indoors working as a physician. Not only had I the patients at the "Humlegaarden," but also a large practice and correspondence out of town; this was more than I could manage.

Organic Gardening Necessary

On January 1st, 1949, I stopped practicing and took up gardening again, which had always been my great interest. For this purpose I had acquired about half a hectare (about one and a quarter acres) of land near the "Humlegaarden," and here I learned how right if was to grow both fruit and vegetables biologically, this is, according to the laws of life. For manure I used only compost, seaweed, straw or hay; no chemical manure, no dung.

In conclusion, just a few words about the practical conditions and the everyday use of raw vegetable food. I am glad to be able to refer to my book "Live Food" which has just been brought out by a Dutch publishing house and which gives a detailed picture of the procedure to be followed to change to a pure raw vegetable diet. It would be of great consequence if the medical profession would acquire greater knowledge in this field to a higher degree than is actually the case. Doctors from Denmark and from foreign countries have visited the "Humlegaarden" for shorter or longer periods of time and have utilized their experience in their practice. The "Humlegaarden" is visited by about one thousand patients annually. Here the patients, as well as the members of the staff, live exclusively on food that has not been treated by heating, and our experience is that a transition diet is quite superfluous. The raw vegetable diet can only be varied according to seasons, and consists of three meals daily. We get a fruit meal in the morning and in the evening and a vegetable meal in the middle of the day. Fruit and vegetables are never mixed. If the condition of the teeth permits it, the raw food is taken whole, otherwise it must be grated and reduced to small particles immediately before the meal. Once the raw food has been grated or chopped, it will not keep because it loses its content of vitamins. The raw food should be carefully chewed, preferably so well that it passes down all by itself, and even the grated raw food should at any rate be mixed well with saliva. All kinds of nuts provide a good supplement. The vegetable meal consists of green leaves, roots and tubers. All fruit is eaten with the peel. In the case of disease such as gastric catarrh, gastric ulcer and the like, care should, however, be taken during the initial stages.

If the exclusively raw food with its associated sound habits of life prevails, a variety of things will improve. Diseases will gradually be obviated. Obesity, the most dangerous of all diseases will become a rarity.

Life a Joy For The Healthy

The housewife's work will be reduced to half the time—and the leisure hours thus gained will be an invaluable advantage and joy for husband, children and home. The slender build, the erect carriage, the supple gait, the fresh complexion, the white, sound teeth and the vigorous hair will dominate the picture. When the body is healthy, the result will invariably be a sound mind. Our negative thoughts will be changed into positive ones and develop the great cultural progress which the world is waiting for. Only then will life be worth living.

MY EXPERIENCE WITH LIVING FOOD

CHAPTER ONE

MY ADOPTION OF A RAW FOOD DIET

That I, a physician, began the consumption of exclusively raw vegetables and fruits was a consequence of a personal illness, a case of cancer of the breast.

As usual, the illness was preceded by a period of poor nutrition and wrong habits, particularly during twelve years of hospital training when I suffered constantly from intestinal stasis and gastric catarrh. At one time I was on the verge of dying of a hemorrhage due to a gastric ulcer.

At this point I dropped meat and fish from my diet, but not until much later did I begin to eat raw vegetables and fruits, increasing the quantity gradually. I obtained a better digestion in this way and was healthier, but I was not yet completely well.

At the end of about ten years of a diet consisting of from fifty to seventy five percent raw vegetables and fruits, although I was unable to diagnose any definite disease. In the spring of 1940, I discovered, quite accidentally, a small tumor in my right breast. But in spite of my fatigue, I disregarded it. Therefore, I was horror-stricken when, five weeks later, I discovered, also accidentally, that this tumor had grown to the size of an egg and had grown into the skin. Only cancer acts in this way.

The usual treatment of cancer is only a makeshift, since we do not know the cause of cancer. I decided at once that I should not submit to that treatment. But what then? I simply had to take some serious steps, otherwise I would soon die of cancer. I felt it almost natural that I should have to live on a 100 percent raw vegetable and fruit diet. With my own life at stake, I was forced to prove the value of a consistent diet of this kind.

I started immediately, going to a small island in the Kattagut, where I lived in a tent, ate raw vegetables exclusively and sunbathed from four to five hours a day when weather permitted. When I felt too warm I plunged into the sea.

My fatigue continued throughout the first two months, and the tumor in my, breast did not diminish. But then my recovery began. The tumor grew smaller as I regained strength, and I felt better than I had for several years.

I had previously consulted the well-known Danish physician Dr. Hindhede, who agreed that I had cancer, but advised me definitely not to submit to a trial microscopy. We both knew that it would open up the blood vessels and cause the cancer to spread. So I gave up that idea.

After I had been feeling normal for about one year on a 100 percent raw vegetable and fruit diet, I adopted Dr. Hindhede's suggestion that I return to my previous diet supplemented by fifty to seventy five percent of raw vegetables. But this proved unsuccessful. In three to four months I began to feel sharp pains in the breast, in the scar tissue left by the tumor at the point where it had originally adhered to the skin. The pains increased in strength during the following weeks, and I suddenly realized that the cancer had become active again! Once again, I returned to the 100 percent raw vegetable and fruit diet, whereupon the pains quickly disappeared as did the fatigue which had preceded the recurrence of the trouble. But on this occasion the cancer was more extensive in the skin of my breast.

What next? I was a physician, so now I had to utilize my experience. My husband and I built a solarium at home large enough to accommodate four or five persons during the next summer. We all ate raw vegetables and fruit, and the patients recovered. Then we sold our house in the suburbs of Copenhagen and bought a property "Humlegaarden," south of Elsinore, where we established a health resort which we have now operated for eleven years.

During these developments the medical authorities began to take notice of my natural treatment for its good results and they did not like it!

And when one of my patients died of diabetes, because he came too late to me, the medical authorities accused me of being responsible for his death, alleging I had not given him enough insulin.

I was promptly called to the court of justice, though a postmortem showed that the patient's liver was in such a condition that it could not function any longer, and that he would have died anyway, even if I had given him more insulin.

The judge and the two jurors—a smith and a farmer—found me guilty and I was ordered not to practice medicine for one year.

If a court were to hold all medical doctors responsible for the deaths of their patients, no doctor would be able to practice.

If I had treated my patients with medicine only and he had died, nothing would have happened to me, but because I was treating my patient with natural methods, I was punished.

Shortly after, I was once more accused on account of the death of two of my patients, one with cancer and the other with tuberculosis. The cancer patient could not follow the living food diet, because of the war when raw fruit and vegetables were very scarce. The tuberculosis patient was living far away from me and I only saw her once; she, too, did not follow the living food diet and died.

Again, I was indicted by my former colleagues for being responsible for the two deaths and once more I was called to the court of justice. This time the jury consisted of two broad minded men, who refused to hold me responsible for the death of two patients. The judge disagreed with the jury and favored the medical doctors so I was found guilty of malpractice.

I could have appealed my case to a higher court, but I was too tired and exhausted fighting single-handedly against my former colleagues who were organized in a strong medical trust.

On the advice of my lawyer I submitted to a compromise arranged by him and the court. I was forced to sign a paper undertaking that I would never practice medicine again in Denmark.

Thus ended completely my treatment of patients with drugs.

Since that time I have been treating all my patients with natural methods, namely by living food, with astonishing results.

My sanatorium "Humlegaarden," always has a waiting list. I do not regret severing my relations with the medical profession, and I am happy to have entered the field of nature cure. Thanks to this persecution by my former colleagues my reputation grew immensely in all Scandinavian countries. This kind of advertisement was worth more to me than money could buy. Thus my former colleagues acted as my free press agents and I have received free publicity in all the Scandinavian newspapers.

During the persecution by the medical doctors I was called a charlatan doctor, but now the doctors have changed their minds about me. They tell their patients who report to them the good results they got in my sanatorium that I am a good psychologist and personage. They do not wish to admit, however, that living food has caused the good results.

I will die, but be sure, living food will live, will be spread all over the whole world and will help to save suffering humanity from all diseases both of body and mind and thereby create one world!

CHAPTER TWO

DETAILS OF THE DIET

How is this consumption of raw vegetables and fruits practiced?
Foods Must Be Properly Combined
Eat Whole Foods Only
Juice Drinking Condemned

We have a meal of fruit in the morning and in the evening and a meal of vegetables at noon. We never eat fruit and vegetables at the same meal. Natural products constitute a unity, in which the component parts are balanced in exact proportion. When separated into juice and dry matter, both parts become one-sided and incomplete. In addition, one could easily drink the juice without salivation and drink more than the gastric juice is able to digest. In short, one would nourish one's disease and not one's health.

Cooked and Dead Foods
Cause Leucocytosis and Leukemia

Here I must mention physiological leucocytosis. The name is derived from "leucocytes," the official name for white blood corpuscles. One cubic millimeter of blood normally contains 6,000—but when we eat dead food, especially sweets and cakes, the number of leucocytes may increase to twice that number, indeed even to three times as much, i.e., to 18,000 per cubic millimeter. And since the leucocytes are the defenders of the organism and always appear where a danger arises, we can understand that the blood becomes strongly poisoned by the dead food we have eaten. Just imagine what a work the production of so many leucocytes in the blood several times a day will impose on an organism. The results may be mortal leukemia.

Consistent consumption of raw vegetables and fruits causes no physiological or digestion leucocytosis.

Cooking Drastically Changes Foods

All fresh, raw vegetables, such as nuts, fruit and vegetables, are basic. But when these things are heated, they all acquire a surplus of acid which is extremely disagreeable to the organism.

Chopped Foods Lose Value Fast

The consumption of raw vegetables and fruits may vary according to season. This is natural and correct. If the teeth are good enough, the raw vegetables and fruit may be simply cleaned and eaten, but if they cannot be chewed well, they must be chopped up finely. They must then be eaten immediately, or 20–25 percent of the vitamins will be lost. Apples may be cut into small pieces, roots and tubers may be grated. Sprouted grain and green leaves may be chopped, but they must not be crushed by passing through a food mincer. Chopped vegetables must be eaten at once, since they wilt rapidly, even under cover. Raw vegetables and fruit must be chewed carefully, preferably until they are virtually a liquid. Even the grated raw vegetables must be mixed with saliva.

With the morning and evening fruit, we eat sprouted rye, sprouted wheat and sprouted yellow peas. Barley and oats take too long to germinate and sour easily. Nuts, especially almonds and coconuts, are the ideal food. The vegetable meal consists of green leaves, roots and tubers. Tomatoes and cucumbers are eaten as vegetables.

Sunshine Is Our Source
For Vitamin D

At "Humlegaarden" we do not use cod liver oil. It is not necessary for Vitamin D. The extremely small quantity of this vitamin required is produced by sunlight on hands and face and can be deposited in the suprarenal glands for use during the winter.

Besides, when we eat raw vegetables and fruits consistently, we preserve a suntanned skin all the year round and perhaps also the ability to produce Vitamin D from the raw vegetables themselves, the live food, the sunlight food. Vegetables contain Vitamin A in abundance.

Foods Are Ideally Organically Grown

The vitamin content of vegetable foods as well as their acid or base-forming capacity, depends greatly on the quality and wholesomeness of the soil from which they are derived. The latter in turn depend on how the soil is treated and fertilized. Therefore tables indicating the vitamin content and acid or alkaline effect of foods are usually contradictory and unreliable.

How do we stand this sudden transition to consistent consumption of raw vegetables? In general we stand it very well.

Raw Food Diet
Sets Off Body Cleansing

To begin with, perhaps even after the first or second meal, the patient gets a headache and symptoms of uric acid poisoning of the organism. He will also experience stomach gas for the first few days. The patients are almost always tired when they arrive, so sufficient rest in the fresh air will be best for them. They must go to bed early with the bedroom windows open. One never feels hungry on a 100 percent raw vegetable and fruit diet, not even when one has lost weight. One does not feel thirsty either.

The Whole Animal Kingdom Is Adapted
To A Raw Food Diet

Will it be possible to work, even to perform hard bodily work on such food? Absolutely. It is easier to work on this diet than on ordinary food, and this applies to both mental and bodily exertion. One feels much better than one has felt for many years on a consistent diet of raw vegetables and fruit. Generally speaking, it is of course, a prerequisite that the organism should be vigorous enough to function, and be able to utilize the raw vegetables and fruit. Sick people often reach understanding of what is needed too late for them to benefit from it.

Why does the consistent use of raw vegetables and fruit have such a good effect on all people?

It has this effect primarily because raw vegetables and fruit are live foods given us by nature. We know, in fact, that all life on the earth is completely dependent on our sun. If we had no sun, the globe would be lifeless, dark and ice-cold. Therefore vitality is synonymous with sun-energy!

However, it is only the plant with its expanse of fine green leaves which is capable of assimilating sunlight and depositing it as roots and tubers, as fruit and seed. We men and animals with solid bodies are incapable of assimilating sunlight directly to the extent required. Therefore both men and animals use plants as intermediaries between themselves and the sun.

Fresh raw vegetable food is life food, sunlight food, the very source of life!

Fresh Raw Fruits and Vegetables Possess Highest Nutritional Values For Mankind

Fresh raw vegetable food, therefore, possesses the highest nutritive value, and this cannot in any way be increased. Drying, withering, storage, fermentation and preservation can only reduce its value. So will boiling, baking or roasting. When life has been removed from the food, its taste disappears. Boiled vegetables have no taste of their own, so something has to be done to them to make them palatable. So we mix together various things, many more than the gastric juices can handle—and add salt, sugar, spices, fat and butter. We remove the germ and the bran from the wheat to make flour for baking. We polish rice, we make artificial sugar from sugar beets; we remove peel, pit and core from apples and pears. We peel potatoes and scrape carrots. We get a large surplus of degenerated animal protein in our food from cooked meat, fish, eggs, cheese, and pasteurized milk. A dangerous thing—surplus albumen cannot be deposited in the organism. What is not needed at once must be removed. And not only does albumen ferment in the digestive organs, but it putrefies and produces foul poisons. We make beverages of coffee, tea, and cocoa beans which contain stimulating poisons which first stimulate the grey cortex of the brain where sensation is coordinated and afterwards paralyze it. We preserve dead foods by means of such poisonous chemicals as benzoic acid, salicylic acid, nitre, boric acid and thiosulfuric acid, in order that it may keep and look well.

Masses Of People Poison Themselves

But not only that! We take pain killers, sleeping draughts, sedatives, laxatives, strong chemical poisons or at any rate substances foreign to the organism. We smoke, inhaling the fumes of poisonous tobacco leaves. Even in small quantities, nicotine is a dangerous poison that weakens the heart. Chronic nicotine poisoning is considered by some American scientists the cause of the heart disease that kills so many busy men at about the age of fifty. Smoking is also the cause of catarrh in the throat, predisposes people to cancer of the throat and lungs, and causes gastric catarrh which can often be corrected only when the patient stops smoking. It tends to make us prematurely old, both internally and externally. Finally, abuse of tobacco is a factor in Burger's disease, the chief symptom of which is gangrene in the feet, often at an early age. Nor should it be forgotten that we cultivate plants incorrectly, spraying our fruit trees with strong chemical poisons, such as lead, arsenic, strychnine and nicotine.

In short, we spoil the raw food, the natural live food, as thoroughly as possible, completely ignorant of the consequences for our health.

Most Foods Now Eaten
Foul The Digestive System

We do not realize or do we understand the profound difference between raw vegetables and fruit on the one hand and ordinary mixed or even vegetarian food on the other hand. The dead food, the carrion food putrefies and ferments in the digestive organs where the temperature is about 98 degrees F. It produces offensive stools and transforms our digestive organs into an evil smelling septic tank. The result is impure blood which gradually leads to a poisoned and weakened organism. On the other hand, raw vegetables and fruit—the live food, the sunlight food—will dissolve and eliminate these poisons. The raw vegetables and fruit are easily digested and produce few waste products. They protect and strengthen the organism in every way, thanks to their content of live, basic vitamins and minerals in their natural combinations.

Vegetarian Animals Admired

Consider the animals. Think of the small Icelandic horse that can run with a man on its back at 6 miles per hour for twelve hours on a rough road. What does it get to eat? Grass, hay and perhaps some oats, but it lives in the open air all year round. Consider the bear! It lives in protected areas on wild berries and honey and can accumulate enough fat to sustain it all winter. It has tremendous strength.

Mankind Despises Carnivores

In contrast think of the carrion-eating animals—jackals, hyenas and vultures—living on dead food. They are ugly, cowardly, weak animals and give off an awful stench. There are about 700,000 different species of animals, all of which, with the exception of the carrion-eating or necrophagous animals, feed on live food. The only other exceptions are men and their domestic animals—the only ones which become ill.

Incorrect Foods Despoiling Mankind

Those who can and will think must be able to understand that our present nutrition is unnatural, devitalized and extremely destructive and is the most serious and general cause of bodily and mental illness and constitutional degeneration. No wonder diseases are rampant! And they are the main causes of economic waste, family and social unrest and war.

We must find the road to healthy nutritional habits if we are to attain prosperity, both now and in the future, and if we hope to succeed in creating one world. We cannot afford to compromise where life and health are concerned. We must follow the only right way—the consistent consumption of raw vegetables and fruit and the simple and natural habits which are the consequence of this diet. It has a curative effect not only for a particular disease and on the individual organ, but on the organism as a whole. It cures not only the disease contracted during our short span of life, but also those determined by hereditary predispositions.

CHAPTER THREE

RESULTS OF THE DIET

What can be obtained through consistent consumption of raw vegetables and fruit?

Improper Diet and Poisons Weaken Our Offspring

In the individual case the result will, on the one hand, depend on how good a constitution the patient has and how old he is, and on the other hand on how poisoned and broken down this constitution has gradually become because of improper nutrition and wrong habits in the past. The embryo growing in a woman can be hurt in two ways. The egg-cell and the sperm cell can determine both bodily and mental disease, but in addition the child may be hurt by the mother's improper nutrition, because it is nourished through the mother's impoverished blood. This may pave the way to disease so that the baby is born ill. After the birth the condition may become aggravated by the fact that the mother's milk may be inadequate in quality and quantity.

All newborn infants throughout the civilized world are born weaklings in some measure, and who can foretell the future consequences thereof?

One "Miracle" of the Living Food Diet

Therefore, the sooner we go in for exclusive consumption of raw vegetables and fruit, the better will be their effect. I shall give an example: A young married couple had eaten 100 percent raw vegetables and fruit for two to three years before they were married. When women do this menstruation ceases, since cleansing is no longer required. As a consequence the young lady did not realize until six weeks before the birth that she was pregnant. By that time she had grown so stout that it could be noticed. She completed labor in about one hour without narcosis and almost without pain. The child was like its mother—small, slight and slender without being skinny—and weighed 5½ pounds. Since the amniotic fluid was scanty the mother's increase in weight immediately before the birth was I I pounds. For this reason she had not felt the new life at the normal time. There had been no room for the child to move around. The mother had abundant milk, so not until the child was three months old did it get mashed fruit after the three breast feedings. The mother gave the breast until the child had enough and felt full. Defecation follows regularly with feeding three times a day. The child never cries unless it is hungry after missing its meal at the regular hour.

Example of a Really Healthy Baby

When the infant in this case was six months old, the mother came and showed it to me. It was small and slight, and though chubby, had not become paunchy. It had one tooth and bit its big toe and thumb alternately; evidently more teeth were developing. The infant was smiling, apparently not afraid of the many people talking loudly in the room. It was given a mashed pear to eat; it could not talk, of course, but it grunted contentedly after each mouthful.

All summer the infant had been in the open air and sunlight most of the day without clothes so that it was nicely suntanned all over. The parents, incidentally, owned a good-sized garden which reduced their food expenditure considerably. Yes, that is the way it ought to be. And it will be so increasingly.

Proper Diet Harmonizes, Not Vitiates, Family life

I have several reports on how a large family of brothers and sisters, living exclusively on raw vegetables and fruits, became sound and happy children in three or four months, and lives in joyful harmony with one another and with society.

So much for the effect of exclusive consumption of raw vegetables and fruits during childhood. The effect on adults cannot be traced so readily but at "Humlegaarden" we certainly obtain strikingly good results in a few weeks, even in the physical field.

Striking Improvement In Well-Being Results From Living Food Diet

Raw vegetables and fruits bring about balance and harmony, kindness and understanding. They can change completely the mentality of the individual. For example, a well-to-do old lady, who was very ill and closefisted, hating to spend money on food for herself or for others, recovered after eating raw vegetables and fruits for some time. She had become kindly and disposed to be helpful. Now all the surplus money she gets is used for aiding others.

A Story of Typical Degeneration on a Conventional Diet and Under Medical Treatment

A woman aged sixty-four had always enjoyed good health up to the age of forty five, when she contracted undulating fever. After the illness she went south to recover. Here she contracted malaria which she had to fight against for several years, during which time she also contracted inflammation of the gall bladder and the biliary ducts, and occasional bronchitis, together with brief lung attacks, phlebitis and anemia.

For five or six years, she suffered from increasing rigidity of the joints, had pneumonia several times, took two x-ray treatments for pain in the back and made several long visits to the hospital.

Finally angina pectoris set in and she had gradually become so stiff and weak that she had to roll out of her bed in the morning. She was unable to fix her hair, being unable to get her hands behind the back of her neck. Her nerves had also gradually degenerated.

Raw Diet Permits Body To Heal Itself

As nothing else could help her, she made up her mind to eat raw vegetables and fruits. She came to "Humlegaarden" and, believe it or not, in about two weeks all her rigidity had disappeared, her movements became free. She had no heart symptoms, and was in high spirits and her nerves were in order. Though I could hardly believe it myself, this result was achieved merely by means of raw vegetables and fruit, fresh air day and night, sun bathing and plenty of rest.

Frugitarian Diet Beneficial For Dogs Too

I have a Doberman Pinscher, a fierce breed of dog, often used for police work. It also feeds on raw vegetables and fruits and is lovableness itself, Although it is eight years old, it appears to be no

CHAPTER FOUR

WEIGHT REDUCTION

The American physiologist, Professor Chittenden, proved by a nine-month nutritional experiment made on himself and twenty-seven other persons —physicians, medical students, soldiers of the ambulance corps and athletes—that people in general eat twice as much as they need.

Proper Weight

A person 5'6" high should not weigh more than about 140 pounds, (with 4 lbs. added for each additional inch. There is no real reason why the weight should be increased as one grows older. On the contrary, the muscles gradually become weaker and weigh less, while the calcium content of the skeleton is reduced with ordinary food and so weighs less. At any rate, weight in later years should not exceed weight in the early adulthood.

Proper Eating Techniques

We must learn to eat slowly, chew well, and avoid over indulgence, by stopping just when the food tastes best. If we still get a feeling of having eaten too much, it is advisable to skip a meal. Then too, we should think of what we eat. By enjoying every mouthful, we increase the flow of gastric juice and thus facilitate digestion. When the feeling of satiety comes, the gastric juice has been used up. If we eat more than the gastric juice can digest, we nourish our diseases instead of our health.

Well chewed food has a great surface relative to quantity and the supply of gastric juice will soon be exhausted. Poorly-chewed food has a much smaller surface in proportion to quantity, so it is necessary to eat more before satiety is experienced.

Dead Food Causes Overeating

Ordinary food, dead food, is so short of vitamins and basic mineral salts that we must eat more calories than are needed in order to get the most necessary of these vitally important substances. This may serve as an explanation and excuse for those who eat too much.

Another explanation is the fact that when by overeating we produce more poisonous waste products than we can eliminate, we must deposit fat in the deep layers of the skin in order to distribute these poisons in such a way that they do the least possible harm to the organism.

Impaired Metabolism Causes Fatness

Finally our organism—our internal glandular system—will gradually deteriorate under continuous overfeeding, so that our metabolic rate is considerably retarded. In this case we will be in worse condition than ever before, because then we must first bring our metabolism back to normal before we can lose weight.

Fatness Indicative of Diseased Body

Excessive adipose tissue is, in fact, nothing less than a poison depot in an over-acid organism. It is for this reason that corpulence is so perilous; it is the starting point for all severe diseases—cancer, arteriosclerosis, rheumatoid arthritis, diabetes, and so on.

Fasting Advised For Fat People

An absolute fasting period with only water compels us to live on our own fat, the poisonous substances contained therein being released into the blood stream and thus eliminated.

Return to Conventional Diet Again Causes Fatness

The first thing the organism will do, when we return again to regular meals is to deposit fat in the deep layers of the skin in order to have the poisonous substances of the blood deposited there. The weight may then increase much more rapidly than when it went down.

It is advisable that one fast until the tongue is clean, by which time all the poisonous substances in the body will have been eliminated.

Raw Diet Also Permits Body To Purify Itself

But, on an exclusive diet of raw vegetables and fruits, it often happens that the tongue becomes heavily coated. At any rate, in the beginning it becomes both yellow and green because of the vastly accelerated elimination of poisoning substances.

It may be readily understood that after uninterrupted fasting for several days, one may feel more active and alive than if one had stuffed himself with the dead food that destroys proper digestion.

The Positive Side of Raw Eating

Naturally, one may also overeat on a diet of raw vegetables and fruits but the temptation is not so great, and the food is automatically chewed better because of its harder composition.

CHAPTER FIVE

THE RAW FOOD DIET IN SPECIFIC CONDITIONS

A well-to-do farmer and his wife had an only daughter of four; they sincerely wished to have more children. I advised them to live on raw vegetables and fruits exclusively, which they did. Three months later the wife was with child, and now they have two more children.

On Nervous Conditions

The diet has a favorable effect on diseases of the automatic nervous system and mental diseases in general, but it takes time—perhaps several years; the same applies to diseases of the internal glandular system such as Basedow's disease. It applies to several serious blood diseases, e.g. pernicious anemia and lymph-ogranulomatosis.

On Diabetes

Consistent consumption of raw vegetables and fruits has a surprisingly beneficial and speedy effect on diabetes, provided the patient has not taken insulin, or, at most, only small quantities of it for a year or two. It helps also when the patient has taken large doses of insulin for several years, but it takes longer; however, even in that case the general condition of the body is rapidly improved.

Overeating a Cause of Diabetes

Raw vegetables and fruits doubtless have such a speedy effect, because in many cases of diabetes it is the increased intake of food which is at fault rather than a decrease in the production of insulin.

Raw vegetables and fruits will reduce food consumption. In addition, several raw vegetables contain insulin, especially Jerusalem artichokes. Most vegetables contain in their raw state the precursor of insulin known as INULIN.

A Generally Ignored Experiment

Five chemists and three physicians in America carried out a protracted examination of four thousand diabetics and concluded that only one percent needed insulin. The rest of them recovered on correct nutrition alone.

Exclusive consumption of raw vegetables and fruits usually makes it easier to break the habits of smoking and drinking. Liquor tastes bad with raw vegetables. In addition, when living on raw vegetables and fruits one craves no stimulants of that kind.

Cancer

Patients suffering from cancer have generally suffered for many years from gastric catarrh and constipation. Cancer is the final stage of pathology in an over-acid and degenerated organism.

If cancer is discovered at an early stage, consistent consumption of raw vegetables and fruits may in many cases keep it in check, even for a considerable number of years. I am a case in point myself. If cancer is discovered at a later stage, consistent consumption of raw vegetables and fruit may certainly help to relieve pain and lengthen life, but it cannot ordinarily preserve life.

Many researchers believe that cancer is a blood disease; once you have it, you will have it for a lifetime. The induration is a local manifestation.

Breast "Cancer" Disappears
On Raw Food Diet

Here I must relate the cases of three patients I had in treatment one summer. The first was a thirty-eight-year-old woman from Malmo, who had an induration the size of a walnut in one breast. She had consulted her doctor, and it had been agreed that an operation should be performed (the breast removed and the armpit cleared).

During the ten days preceding the operation she stayed at "Humlegaarden," and lived exclusively on raw vegetables and fruits. On her return she consulted her doctor. It was discovered that the induration was by this time the size of a grain of rice, so she escaped the operation. The patient is still living exclusively on raw vegetables and fruits, and has reduced her weight by 22 lbs., looks ten years younger and feels better than she has felt for many years.

Breast Operations Criminal

The second case was a woman of forty-nine. She stayed with me for some time before she discovered an induration the size of a large nut in her breast. She became horror-stricken. I proposed that she stay with me and see what raw vegetables and fruits could do for her, but fear drove her to a doctor in the neighborhood, who told her; "You must go back to Bergen to have an operation at once."

She asked him whether he believed raw vegetables and fruit could help her, and he answered that he would wager his head they would not. Nevertheless, the patient decided to stay with me for two weeks. After six days she asked me to take a look at the induration. I found it but it was now the size of a pin head.

On the following day she went to the doctor she had called on before. He examined her and exclaimed: "What have you not gone yet?" And she answered that she would like to have the induration examined before she left. "And then," she said to me, "You should have seen him gape when he could not find it. " One should be careful not to wager one's head on things one does not know about!

The third case was a Swedish woman of sixty two with a nut sized induration in her breast. It decreased to a pea size during the four weeks she stayed with me. And three weeks later she wrote me that it had disappeared.

I have had several other examples of patients with cancer discovered microscopically or (as in the case of cancer in the stomach) in the course of a futile operation, who have recovered or are, at any rate alive and able to work.

The treatment has been applied to cancer of the rectum, of the large intestine, of the abdomen, of the stomach and to a single case of a primary pulmonary tumor, which was probably cancer.

Another Illustrative Case History

Another example is that of a Swedish woman in her forties who had been ill for six years suffering from increasingly severe pains in the back of her neck and head. During the last four years her vision declined and her head buzzed, impairing her hearing. The faculty of feeling in most of the upper part of body, especially in the fingertips, began to decline for short periods, then almost continually. At the same time the pains in her head and the back of her neck had become so violent that she would lie on the floor in convulsions.

The patient came to me from "Skodsborg Sanitorium" where she had spent two months without improvement. Her doctor had told her that she was well and could return to her home. With her last remnants of energy she came to "Humlegaarden," where I received her —sick and miserable as she was. I had to try to help her!

When she had been with me for a couple of weeks, I gathered from the symptoms that there must be a tumor in her cerebellum, pressing on the optic nerve, the aural nerve and the sensory nerves of the upper part of her body. I told her so, adding that I would attempt to help her, if she herself had the courage. Not till then did I learn that she had consulted a Swedish specialist on diseases of the brain who said she had an inoperable cerebral tumor.

She stayed with me for four months and recovered—completely, one may say, inasmuch as all the symptoms had disappeared. This does not mean to say, however, that the tumor had vanished entirely but it had at any rate been reduced so much in size that it no longer pressed on the nerves as before. If the patient continues in Sweden with raw vegetables and fruits, I believe the tumor will disappear completely. It was probably not cancer but a glioma, or slowly growing form of tumor, found only in the brain, but so virulent that it may reappear if the patient forsakes the raw vegetables and fruits.

A Warning

One thing I must urgently warn against is a biopsy or microscopic examination of tissue for cancer. I had it performed on myself in January, 1948 because so many physicians said that I never had cancer. This biopsy was made by the "Radium-station" in Copenhagen and it was positive. There were cancer cells in the scar tissue in the skin on my breast but it was the most benign form in existence, the one called scirrhus. My rapidly growing and previously virulent cancerous tumor had been converted under the influence of raw vegetables and fruits into the most benign form in existence.

Nevertheless, this operation nearly gave cancer the upper hand, so I became fearful. For the first time I had a secondary growth in the armpit in the shape of two nut sized indurations. The cancer spread widely in the skin of my breast. It took me six months to calm down. Since then I have been all right!

It was more that I could manage. In January, 1949 I gave up my practice. All patients coming to "Humlegaarden" know actually what their illness is. They have consulted specialists and visited hospitals. Here they need only information about the use of raw vegetables and fruits.

Sunshine a Great Benefit To Health

We have a fine garden for sunbathing at "Humlegaarden." It is sheltered and open to the south, so that both men and women may bathe in the sun unclothed. Supervised sunbathing is itself a great remedy. Our patients are fortified by the diet against the more intense rays of the sun.

Fresh Air Most Important

I have frequently to remind the patients that fresh air is a part of our nutrition—perhaps the most important part. We can fast for weeks, but we can do without air for only two minutes. Since we use five or six hundred quarts of air per hour we can soon exhaust the oxygen in a small room whose windows and doors are closed.

We then inhale our own exhaled carbon dioxide and awaken to a heavy head in the morning. Clean fresh air is plentiful at Oresund, so we keep the windows open at night! Warm bedclothes make it easy for those with rheumatism and other chronic diseases to accept this regimen.

In summer we can accommodate twenty five patients in semi-open cabins, which are perfect for sound sleep.

Most patients arrive with constipation; defecation returns to normal through an exclusive diet of raw vegetables, and fruits.

A Home Garden Advisable

We must attempt to provide each family with a house of its own and a garden large enough for growing fruits, roots and green vegetables in the proper way. They should not be stored before using.

Ravi, Diet Saves Much Work

When housewives introduce raw vegetables and fruits into the daily diet, they are relieved of hours of cooking and then use the time saved for gardening.

Gardening Has Immense Side Benefits

Nobody can avoid manual work, and there is no better form of it than gardening. Carried on in fresh air it is the most many sided form of exercise—superior to sport—which puts every muscle to work. "By the sweat of thy brow shalt thou eat bread," is still applicable. Here I would call attention to an old Chinese proverb: Life begins on the day you start a garden.

Proper Life Style Begets Marvelous Results

I assure you that it is a great delight to survey all that can be grown in the ground: nuts, fruit, vegetables and flowers. Men, women and children become strong, healthy and happy persons, eager to help others.

An erect carriage, lithe figure, easy gait, fresh skin, sparkling eyes, live strong hair, white strong teeth, and a warm, heart winning smile are more beautiful than anything ever dreamed of by hairdressers or cosmeticians.

Heart Weakness

When the arteries calcify, they become stiff and thick-walled. Since the space inside is reduced, the blood pressure increased, the work of the heart is increased, the heart muscles become stronger, and the heart becomes a hard muscle. But, with the gradual increase of arteriosclerosis, the heart can no longer perform its task. It becomes gradually an atonic bag, with the result that blood pressure declines and may fall far below normal.

Too high as well as too low blood pressure involves a slow circulation of the blood, so that it carries less nourishment to the organism and removes less waste, leaving the organism undernourished and poisoned. The sufferer feels cold, —specially in the hands and feet, even when wearing extra clothes. If, in addition, the vessels nourishing the heart itself are calcified, the patient gets angina pectoris, agonizing heart attacks, which may result in heart failure and death.

Heart Normalizes to the Extent Possible on Proper Diet

If the patient gets raw vegetables and fruit at this point, the heart will be strengthened and will function better, while the blood pressure may increase regardless of whether it is already too high or too low. Often the patient does not understand this, and becomes fearful, but if only he will be patient, the excessively high blood pressure will fall to normal (about 120–125) with consistent consumption of raw vegetables and fruit.

CHAPTER SIX

The Importance of Mineral Salts

All our diseases, ranging from cancer and heart diseases, the two most frequent causes of death, to fatigue and sleeplessness, are the result of improper nourishment and unhygienic living habits.

Even in America one is often invited to support foundations for curing cancer, infantile paralysis, rheumatism and so on. Or one may read statistics reporting that 98 percent of American children have decayed teeth, that out of five, four are undernourished, and that almost all of them have colds.

Some Nutritional Roles of Mineral Salts

It is recognized that out of almost one hundred mineral salts, at least sixteen are indispensable for our organism and several others are to be found in our organism, although their precise physiological role has not yet been established. Among the most important indispensable salts are calcium, phosphorus and iron. Calcium regulates the activity of the nerves, so it is extremely important for the generation of cells in all living creatures. It controls muscular contractions and the rhythmic pulsation of the heart. It cooperates with other mineral salts and adjusts disturbances caused by them. It always acts in cooperation with vitamin D.

Calcium Deficiency Widespread In America

But half the American people suffer from lack of calcium. At a hospital in New York only two out of four thousand patients had enough of the element.

What does such a shortage mean? How will it influence your health and mine? Well, the result is so many cases of poor health and actual diseases that it is almost hopeless to enumerate them. Rickets, decayed teeth, reduced resistance to other diseases, fatigue and lack of adaptability are some of the most significant.

Here is a specific case. The soil of an area in the midwest of the United States, is short of calcium. When three hundred children from that area were examined, almost ninety percent had decayed teeth. Sixty-nine percent had nose-catarrh and pharyngitis, swollen glands and enlarged and inflamed tonsils, while more than one-third of these children had weak vision, round shoulders, bandy legs and anemia.

Raw vegetables are our best source of calcium. Phosphorus and calcium seem to cooperate. A child's daily need for this mineral equals that of two adult men. Examination of our ordinary food shows a general shortage of calcium and phosphorus.

Shortage of iron causes anemia. Yet iron cannot be absorbed unless the food also contains copper. In Florida many cattle die of a disease called "salt disease," which is due to insufficient iron and copper in the soil.

If our food does not contain iodine, the thyroid gland cannot function with the result that tumor or goiter develops. Although the human organism must have only one-fourteen thousands milligram of iodine per day, diseases caused from deficiency of it are found in certain areas of Europe and America.

Vitamin B12 Formed in Body If Cobalt Present

If there is no cobalt to form vitamin B_{12}, pernicious anemia will be the consequence. And so the list continues. Every mineral salt plays its role in nutrition. Characteristic symptoms, as specific as the actual diseases caused by shortage of vitamins, accompany each of these valuable health promoting substances. We might be tempted to say, "Well, if our food is so destitute of these mineral salts, why not resort to drugs?"

Mineral Salts Assimilable Only From Organic Sources

This is just what is now often attempted. However, those who know assure us that we cannot absorb these substances to advantage in anything but food. I would even specify living food. They cannot be absorbed in the form of medicine. Apart from phosphorus and calcium, they are only required in infinitely small quantities, and the effect of one of them may depend on the presence of another.

Soil Depletion of Minerals a Problem

This is a very serious problem, but nature both can and will solve it. We can help her to do so. Mineral salts in fruits and vegetables are colloidal, which means that they are in a state of such extreme suspension that they can be absorbed in the human organism. It is merely a question of giving back to nature the materials which she works with.

We must restore our soil; we must restore to it the mineral salts we have taken from it through plants. It may seem difficult but it is not. This is, in short, the way to better health and longer life.

When we first learned that a great part of our food lacked mineral salts and that this deficiency was to be ascribed to shortage of these elements in the soil, we laughed at those who were foolish enough to believe it. But difference of opinion in medical science is nothing new. Textbooks cannot be trusted, since many of the analyses are obsolete, based perhaps on products raised in virgin soil, while our soil has gradually been exhausted. Soil analyses are samples. One analysis may be quite different from another taken a few miles away.

Soil Replenishment Easy

But what could be done about it? Experiments were made which proved that a good soil-balance in respect to mineral salts (obtained by use of crushed rock) yields crops that contain the mineral salts desired. In addition, it will be proved that crops raised on mineralized soil are both larger and better, that grain germinates and grows more rapidly and yields better plants, that the trees become more sturdy and bear more fruit of a better quality.

By increasing the mineral content of the soil in the lemon groves, sweeter fruits with a finer aroma and better quality are obtained.

Sick soil means sick plants which are like feeble, underfed, anemic children.

A sound plant growing on sound soil can endure most diseases, which means that it becomes better food for men. Almost everyone is a host both for tuberculosis and pneumonia germs, but these bacilli are impotent against a healthy physical condition. Similarly, a plant becomes strong in its natural struggles and thus is made more suitable for the satisfaction of human needs.

What does this mean to agriculture? It means perfect food, better crops, and lower costs of living.

We may put an end to our liability to infection by providing ourselves with food which contains the mineral salts our organism requires. This immunity is the only one humans and animals can have. Patent medicines and inoculations cannot establish immunity.

No one really knows his own physical or mental capacity, however well he may feel or however long he may live, because at the present time we are all cripples and weaklings. But we shall be on the way towards better health if we restore to the soil the mineral salts and humus which have been taken from it.

Here in Denmark our rock-meal comes from the blue granite or limestone bedrock of Bornholm. I have now used blue granite for three years. I discovered that during the first year it is used it will have no effect, for it must have time to erode a little. These observations about its effect apply to northern fruits and vegetables. But experiments have demonstrated that basalt, a black igneous rock, and copper ore are still better.

Artificial Fertilizers Harmful to Soil and Produce Deficient Foods

We could get basalt from all parts of Iceland, since the whole island is covered by a heavy layer of lava. The bedrock there has not yet been reached. We could get copper ore from Norway, where it exists in large quantities, and from other places where the ore is of such low grade that it does not pay to extract the copper. It would make a good fertilizer. In both Iceland and Norway electric power is available for pulverizing rock. Let us abandon artificial manure. It makes the soil sour, discourages earthworms, kills the bacteria of the soil and makes the surface crusty in dry weather.

If Iceland and Norway utilized their minerals by grinding them into fertilizer, they would greatly enrich the soil. This step is bound to come soon. We cannot afford to wait longer, now that we have the knowledge.

CHAPTER SEVEN

CONCLUSION

Finally, we all remember from the serious losses we have suffered that time heals all wounds. How often has personal loss seemed, at a proper distance, for all the best. If all things went as we wished them, life would indeed be uninteresting.

Hence ideals of a kind are essential. If we possess an ideal, however modest it may be, and pursue it vigilantly, then everything will make for progress and success. A high ideal, merely professed, will lead us from one failure to another and we shall reap as we have sown. Nature herself is merciless, knowing nothing of compassion. But when we are sick, tired, dull and morally defective, we sometimes try to take short cuts. Even though we are misled by them, we still like to keep our old habits. Pills, for example, are usually mere chemical poisons, but they are familiar and easy to take. They have no relation to the cause of disease, although they do affect the symptoms, narcotize the organism so that it cannot function, and add new poisons to those already present.

But if today's resolution fails, we must reaffirm it tomorrow—but never cease to make the effort.

If by means of raw vegetables and fruits, we can become so mentally strong and healthy that our innermost conviction may be followed, then surely all is well.

DISTRIBUTION OF VITAMINS IN RAW VEGETABLES AND FRUITS

VITAMIN A

As carotene or Provitamin A

(1) in green leaves, e.g. cabbage and lettuce.

(2) in yellowish and red fruits and vegetables, e.g. oranges, rose hips; raspberries, tomatoes and carrots.

The stronger the green or red color, the greater the content of carotene.

VITAMIN B

The vitamin B complex is a variety of related vitamins, almost always existing together. We know of vitamins B_1 to B_{17}.

Foodstuffs rich in the B vitamin are:

All nuts, most vegetables, especially lettuce, Brussels sprouts, cabbage, kale, and legumes such as peas, peanuts, beans and alfalfa.

VITAMIN C

Vitamin C exists in all fresh vegetables and fruits, particularly in:

Brussels sprouts, kale, cabbage, cauliflower, lettuce and bell pepper. Rose hips, black currants, strawberries, lemons, oranges, grapefruit and limes.

VITAMIN D

Our best Vitamin D source is sunshine. Sunflower seeds are the best vegetable source.

VITAMIN E

Vitamin E is to be found in the embryo of most seeds, (especially of sunflower seeds) green plants, especially lettuce. green peas and beans.

We'd love to send you a free catalog of titles we publish
or even hear your thoughts, reactions, criticism,
about things you did or didn't like about this
or any other book we publish.

Just write or call us at:

TEACH Services, Inc.
254 Donovan Road
Brushton, New York 12916-9738
1-800-367-1998

http://www.teachservicesinc.com